One-M

Unlock the Secret to Healing Doctors Never Learned

Author: **Aniya Tyler**

All rights reserved @Copyright 2025.

Without the express, explicit permission of the author and/or publisher, no part of this book may be reproduced, transmitted, or copied in any form whatsoever.

Neither the book's publisher nor the author will be held liable for any losses or injuries, financial or otherwise, that may occur as a direct or indirect result of following.

Notice of Legal Effects:

This book is subject to copyright regulations. For your eyes only, if you will. The content may not be modified, copied, sold, used, quoted, or paraphrased in any way without the prior written consent of the author or publisher.

Disclaimer Notice:

Please note that this document is intended for educational and informational purposes only. Every effort has been made to ensure the information is as accurate, current, reliable, and comprehensive as possible. However, the content in this book is derived from various natural herbal sources. If you do not fully understand any of the strategies mentioned, please consult us via email for further clarification before using them.

By using this information, whether or not it contains errors or inaccuracies, you acknowledge that the author is not liable for any direct or indirect damages resulting from your reliance on the content provided.

ISBN: 978-1-300-67326-2

Author: Aniya Tyler

Book Title: One-Minute Cure: Unlock the Secret to Healing Doctors Never Learned

TABLE OF CONTENTS

INTRODUCTION — 1

HERBAL REMEDIES — 2

HERBAL TEAS FOR HIGH BLOOD PRESSURE (HYPERTENSION) — 2

HERBAL TEAS FOR HYPOTENSION - LOW BLOOD PRESSURE — 4

HERBAL TEA RECIPES FOR ACUTE BRONCHITIS — 4

HERBAL TEAS FOR BRONCHIAL CATARRH — 5

HERBAL TEAS FOR BURNS — 6

HERBAL TEA RECIPES FOR COMMON COLD — 7

HERBAL TEAS FOR CONJUNCTIVITIS — 10

HERBAL TEAS FOR CONSTIPATION — 10

HERBAL TEA RECIPES FOR COUGH — 13

HERBAL TEA RECIPES WHOOPING COUGH — 18

HERBAL TEA RECIPES FOR CYSTITIS — 20

HERBAL TEAS FOR DIABETES — 21

HERBAL TEAS FOR IMPOTENCE — 23

HERBAL TEA RECIPES FOR INDIGESTION   24

HERBAL TEAS FOR INSOMNIA   27

HERBAL TEA RECIPES FOR JAUNDICE   30

HERBAL TEAS FOR KIDNEY STONES   33

HERBAL RECIPES FOR LACTATION DISORDERS   35

HERBAL TEAS FOR LARYNGITIS   38

HERBAL TEAS FOR LEUCORRHOEA   39

HERBAL TEA RECIPES FOR MENSTRUAL DISORDERS 40

HERBAL TEA RECIPES FOR NAUSEA   43

HERBAL TEAS FOR NERVOUS EXHAUSTION   45

HERBAL TEA RECIPES FOR NEURALGIA   46

HERBAL TEA RECIPES FOR DROPSY   48

HERBAL TEA RECIPES FOR PHLEBITIS & VARICOSE VEINS   50

HERBAL TEA RECIPES FOR PILES   51

HERBAL TEA RECIPES FOR ENLARGED PROSTATE GLAND   53

HERBAL TEAS FOR SKIN DISORDERS   56

HERBAL TEA RECIPES FOR BLOOD IN THE URINE   57

HERBAL TEA RECIPES FOR PAINFUL URINATION (DYSURIA)   57

HERBAL TEA RECIPES FOR VOMITING   59

HERBAL TEA RECIPES FOR WOUNDS   61

INTRODUCTION

For centuries, traditional medicine has relied on herbal remedies, providing a natural and holistic approach to health and well-being. Ancient civilizations and modern-day communities harness the healing power of plants to treat a wide array of ailments. Today, we see a resurgence in interest and practice of herbal medicine, as these natural therapies gain recognition for their safety, effectiveness, and sustainability.

Herbal remedies serve as essential treatments, forming a crucial part of a vast body of knowledge that generations have passed down. Herbalists, healers, and cultural practices around the world provide wisdom, with each plant offering unique properties and benefits. As the world of pharmaceuticals grows, more individuals turn to herbs to enhance their health, address chronic conditions, or find balance in their lives.

This book provides a comprehensive guide to understanding herbal remedies and showcases the vast potential of plants in promoting wellness. As a seasoned herbalist or a newcomer, you will gain practical, accessible, and scientifically supported knowledge on incorporating herbs into your daily life. Discover how specific plants aid in digestion, boost immunity, reduce stress, support mental clarity, and more. Herbs provide healing properties that create an exciting opportunity to explore nature's medicine cabinet and take charge of your health.

This book explores the art and science of using herbs for healing, respecting both ancient traditions and modern research. This guide presents information in an approachable yet professional tone, helping you confidently incorporate herbal remedies into your lifestyle. This guide helps you identify common herbs and understand their safe and effective uses, unlocking the natural benefits that herbs offer.

Research increasingly validates the therapeutic potential of herbal remedies, prompting us to rediscover and embrace these time-tested treatments. Explore the incredible healing potential of the plant kingdom and gain a deeper understanding of how to cultivate health, prevent disease, and restore balance in your life. Join us on this journey as we explore herbal remedies and reconnect with the Earth's wisdom.

HERBAL REMEDIES

Herbal Teas for High Blood Pressure (Hypertension)

Recipe #1: Alfalfa Seed Tea
Ingredients:

- 1 teaspoon crushed Alfalfa seeds
- 4 cups water

Preparation:
Boil the Alfalfa seeds in 4 cups of water for 30 minutes. Strain the mixture.
Preparation time: 30 minutes
Dosage: Drink 1 cup of tea, 6-7 times a day.

Recipe #2: Hawthorn Blossom and Leaf Tea
Ingredients:

- 1 teaspoon crushed dried Hawthorn blossoms
- 1 teaspoon crushed dried Hawthorn leaves
- 1 cup boiling water

Preparation:
Combine the Hawthorn blossoms, leaves, and boiling water in a suitable container. Cover and allow the mixture to steep for 20 minutes. Strain the tea.
Preparation time: 20 minutes
Dosage: Drink ½ cup of tea, 2-3 times a day.

Recipe #3: Marigold Flower Tea
Ingredients:

- 1-2 teaspoons crushed Marigold flower heads
- 2 cups boiling water

Preparation:
Add the crushed Marigold flowers to the boiling water and let them steep for 15-20 minutes. Discard the flowers, and the tea is ready to drink.
Preparation time: 15-20 minutes
Dosage: Drink 1 cup of tea, twice a day.

Recipe #4: Parsley Tea
Ingredients:

- 1 teaspoon chopped Parsley
- 1 cup water

Preparation:
Place the chopped Parsley into 1 cup of water, bring it to a boil, then remove from heat. Let the tea sit for 15 minutes, then strain.
Preparation time: 15 minutes
Dosage: Drink 1 tablespoon several times a day.

Recipe #5: Red Periwinkle Tea
Ingredients:

- 1 teaspoon crushed fresh or sun-dried Red Periwinkle leaves
- 1 cup water

Preparation:
Suspend the crushed Red Periwinkle leaves in the water and bring it to a boil. Cover and simmer for 10 minutes, then remove from heat and strain.
Preparation time: 10 minutes
Dosage: Drink 1 tablespoon of tea once a day.

Recipe #6: Stinging Nettle Tea
Ingredients:

- 1 handful chopped young Stinging Nettle leaves
- 2 cups boiling water

Preparation:
Mix the chopped Stinging Nettle leaves into the boiling water. Cover and steep for 15 minutes, then strain. For added flavor, a little lemon juice can be added.
Preparation time: 15 minutes
Dosage: Drink ¼ cup of tea once a day.

Herbal Teas for Hypotension – Low Blood Pressure

Rosemary Tea
Ingredients:

- 1 teaspoon crushed fresh or dried Rosemary leaves
- 1 cup boiling water

Preparation:
Place the crushed Rosemary leaves in a suitable container and pour the boiling water over them. Cover the container and allow the tea to steep for 5 to 10 minutes. Strain the tea and serve.
Preparation time: 5-10 minutes
Dosage: Drink 1 cup, twice a day.

Herbal Tea Recipes for Acute Bronchitis

Herbal Tea for Acute Bronchitis #1

Ingredients:

- 1–2 teaspoons of finely chopped Elecampane root
- 2 ½ cups of water

Preparation: Boil the chopped Elecampane root in water for 15 to 20 minutes. Once the boiling is complete, remove the mixture from heat and let it steep for 15 minutes. Afterward, strain and enjoy.

Preparation Time: 15–20 minutes of boiling, plus 15 minutes of steeping
Dosage: Drink 1 cup twice daily.

Herbal Remedy for Acute Bronchitis #2

Ingredients:

- 1 handful of dried Horehound flowering plant, ground
- 2 cups of water

Preparation: Bring the Horehound and water mixture to a boil. Remove from heat and allow it to steep for 20 minutes. Once cooled, strain the mixture and drink.

Preparation Time: 20 minutes
Dosage: Consume 1 cup per day, taking 1 tablespoon at a time.

Herbal Teas for Bronchial Catarrh

Herbal Tea for Bronchial Catarrh #1

Ingredients:

- 1 tablespoon of crushed Aniseed seeds
- 2 cups of water

Preparation: Combine the crushed Aniseed seeds and water in a covered pan and bring to a boil. Once boiled, remove from heat, allow it to cool, strain, and enjoy.

Preparation Time: 1 minute
Dosage: Drink 1 cup twice daily.

Herbal Tea for Bronchial Catarrh #2

Ingredients:

- 1 tablespoon of dried Pine young shoots
- 1 cup of water

Preparation: Soak the Pine herb in cold water, then bring the mixture to a boil. Once boiling, remove from heat and let it steep, covered, for 15 minutes. Strain the mixture before drinking.

Preparation Time: 1-2 minutes of boiling, 15 minutes of steeping
Dosage: Drink ½ cup twice daily.

Herbal Teas for Burns

Herbal Tea Recipes for Burns #1

Ingredients:

- 1-2 teaspoons of crushed Marigold flower heads
- 2 cups of boiling water

Preparation:
Place the crushed Marigold flowers in a pan, cover with boiling water, and steep for 15 minutes with the lid on. Strain the mixture and drink.

Preparation Time: 15 minutes
Dosage: 1 cup per day

Herbal Tea Recipes for Burns #2

Ingredients:

- 2 teaspoons of crushed Stinging Nettle dried leaves
- 1 cup of water

Preparation:
Boil the Stinging Nettle leaves and water for 5 minutes. Remove from the heat, cover, and let it steep for 1 hour. Strain and drink.

Preparation Time: 5 minutes of boiling; 1 hour of steeping
Dosage: ½ cup, three times a day

Herbal Tea Recipes for Common Cold

Herbal Tea Recipes for Common Cold #1

Ingredients:

- 3g of powdered Cinnamon bark
- 1 ½ cups of water

Preparation:
Boil the Cinnamon bark in water for 15 minutes in a covered container. Strain and sweeten with sugar, if desired, before drinking.

Preparation Time: 15 minutes
Dosage: ½ cup, twice a day

Herbal Tea Recipes for Common Cold #2

Ingredients:

- 2 teaspoons of dried Dog Rose rose hips, shredded
- 2 cups of water

Preparation:
Boil the shredded Dog Rose in water for 10 minutes, keeping the pot covered. Strain the mixture and drink twice a day.

Preparation Time: 10 minutes
Dosage: 1 cup, twice a day

Herbal Teas for Common Cold #3

Ingredients:

- 30g of shredded Ginger rhizomes
- 2 cups of boiling water

Preparation:
Cover the shredded Ginger rhizomes with boiling water, cover the pan, and steep for 5-20 minutes depending on the strength you prefer. Strain and drink.

Preparation Time: 5-20 minutes
Dosage: 1-2 cups per day

Herbal Tea Recipes for Common Cold #4

Ingredients:

- 1 teaspoon of dried Holy Basil leaves, crushed
- 2 cups of water

Preparation:
Boil the crushed Holy Basil leaves in 2 cups of water until only 1 cup of liquid remains. Strain the mixture and discard the leaves.

Preparation Time: 15 minutes
Dosage: 2 tablespoons, four times a day

Herbal Teas for Common Cold #5

Ingredients:

- 1 teaspoon of powdered Liquorice
- ½ cup of boiling water

Preparation:
Mix the powdered Liquorice in ½ cup of boiling water. Let it sit for 5 minutes before straining. Drink after meals.

Preparation Time: 5 minutes
Dosage: ½ cup, three times a day after meals

Herbal Recipes for Common Cold #6

Ingredients:

- 6g of fresh Flower petals, crushed
- 1 ½ cups of water

Preparation:
Add the crushed flowers to the water, bring to a boil for 15 minutes, keeping the container covered. Strain and discard the flowers.

Preparation Time: 15 minutes
Dosage: ½ cup, twice a day

Herbal Teas for Common Cold #7

Ingredients:

- 1 teaspoon of dried or fresh whole Plant, chopped
- 1 cup of boiling water

Preparation:
Soak the herb in the boiling water for 5-10 minutes, then strain and drink.

Preparation Time: 5-10 minutes
Dosage: 1 cup, three times a day

Herbal Teas for Conjunctivitis

Ingredients:

- 1 tablespoon of dried Eyebright herb, crushed
- 1 cup of water

Preparation:
Stir the crushed Eyebright into the water, bring it to a boil for 2 minutes. Remove from heat, cover, and cool for 5-10 minutes. Strain before use.

Preparation Time: 2 minutes boiling, 5-10 minutes standing
Dosage: 1 cup, three times a day

Herbal Teas for Constipation

Herbal Teas for Constipation #1

Ingredients:

- 6 Chebulic Myrobalan fruits, crushed
- 1 ¼ cups of water

Preparation:
Boil the crushed Chebulic Myrobalan fruits with 3g of cinnamon in water for 10 minutes. Strain and drink in the morning.

Preparation Time: 10 minutes
Dosage: ½ cup, once a day

Herbal Teas for Constipation #2

Ingredients:

- 1 teaspoon of crushed Fennel seeds
- ½ cup of water

Preparation:
Soak the crushed Fennel seeds in water for 30 minutes, keeping the container covered. Strain and drink.

Preparation Time: 30 minutes
Dosage: 1 teaspoon, twice a day

Herbal Tea Recipes for Constipation #3

Ingredients:

- 12g of Purging Cassia pulp from ripe pods
- ½ cup of boiling water

Preparation:
Pour boiling water over the Purging Cassia pulp and let it sit uncovered for 5-6 hours. Strain and drink before bed.

Preparation Time: 5-6 hours
Dosage: 1 tablespoon, at bedtime

Home Made Herbal Tea Recipes for Constipation #4

Ingredients:

- 1 teaspoon of crushed Senna leaves
- 1 cup of boiling water

Preparation:
Steep the crushed Senna leaves in boiling water for 30 minutes, keeping the lid on. Strain and drink before bed.

Preparation Time: 30 minutes
Dosage: ½ cup, at bedtime

Herbal Teas for Constipation #5

Ingredients:

- 1/3 teaspoon of powdered Fennel seeds
- 1/3 teaspoon of powdered Linseed seeds
- 1/3 teaspoon of powdered Liquorice root
- 1 ¾ cups of water

Preparation:
Mix equal parts of the three herbs, add to the water, and boil for 10 minutes, keeping the pot covered. Strain the decoction and drink.

Preparation Time: 10 minutes
Dosage: 1 cup, three times a day

Herbal Tea Recipes for Cough

Herbal Tea Recipes for Cough #1

Ingredients:

- 1-2 teaspoons of crushed Aniseed seeds
- 1 cup of boiling water

Preparation:
Place the crushed Aniseed seeds in a pan, pour over boiling water, cover, and let it steep for 15 minutes. Strain and drink while hot.

Preparation Time: 15 minutes
Dosage: 1 cup, 2-3 times a day

Herbal Tea Recipes for Cough #2

Ingredients:

- 14g of ground Catnip leaves and flowering tops
- 2 cups of boiling water

Preparation:
Pour boiling water over the Catnip herb and steep for 5-10 minutes. Strain and drink at room temperature.

Preparation Time: 5-10 minutes
Dosage: 1 cup in the morning and 1 cup at bedtime
Caution: Not recommended for children under two years old

Herbal Tea Recipes for Cough #3

Ingredients:

- ½ teaspoon of crushed Eucalyptus leaves
- 2/3 cup of boiling water

Preparation:
Steep the Eucalyptus leaves in boiling water for 20 minutes. Keep the pot covered. Strain and drink.

Preparation Time: 20 minutes
Dosage: 2/3 cup, three times a day

Herbal Recipes for Cough #4

Ingredients:

- 1 handful of crushed Horehound flowering tops
- 2 cups of water

Preparation:
Boil the Horehound in 2 cups of water for 15 minutes, covered. Let it stand for an additional 15 minutes, strain, and drink at room temperature.

Preparation Time: 15 minutes boiling, 15 minutes standing
Dosage: 1 cup per day, 1 tablespoon at a time

Herbal Recipes for Cough #5

Ingredients:

- 15g of crushed Linseed seeds
- 2 cups of boiling water

Preparation:
Pour boiling water over the crushed Linseed seeds, cover, and steep for 5-20 minutes. Strain and drink hot or warm.

Preparation Time: 5-20 minutes
Dosage: 1-2 cups per day

Herbal Tea Recipes for Cough #6

Ingredients:

- 7 Malabar Nut leaves, crushed
- 1 cup of boiling water

Preparation:
Steep the crushed Malabar Nut leaves in boiling water for 15 minutes, covered. Strain and drink.

Preparation Time: 15 minutes
Dosage: 1-4 tablespoons, four times a day

Herbal Teas for Cough #7

Ingredients:

- 1-2 teaspoons of chopped Violet dried flowers
- 2 cups of boiling water

Preparation:
Place the chopped Violet flowers in boiling water, steep for 5-7 minutes, strain, and drink while still warm.

Preparation Time: 5-7 minutes
Dosage: 1 cup, three times a day

Herbal Recipes for Cough #8

Ingredients:

- 2-3 teaspoons of crushed Yarrow dried flowering plant
- 4 cups of cold water

Preparation:
Infuse the Yarrow in cold water, allowing the mixture to stand for 6-8 hours. Strain before drinking.

Preparation Time: 6-8 hours
Dosage: 1 cup, four times a day

Herbal Teas for Cough #9

Ingredients:

- ¼ teaspoon of powdered Coltsfoot leaves
- ¼ teaspoon of powdered Comfrey leaves
- ¼ teaspoon of powdered Marshmallow root
- ¼ teaspoon of powdered Sage leaves
- 2 cups of boiling water

Preparation:
Combine the powdered herbs, pour boiling water over them, and let the mixture steep, covered, for 15 minutes. Strain and drink.

Preparation Time: 15 minutes
Dosage: 1 cup, three times a day

Herbal Tea Recipes for Cough #10

Ingredients:

- 1/3 teaspoon of powdered Aniseed
- 1/3 teaspoon of powdered Sundew whole plant
- 1/3 teaspoon of powdered Thyme whole plant
- 1 cup of boiling water

Preparation:
Combine the herbs, pour over boiling water, cover, and steep for 15 minutes. Strain and drink.

Preparation Time: 15 minutes
Dosage: 1 cup, three times a day

Home Made Herbal Tea Recipes for Cough #11

Ingredients:

- 3g of powdered Liquorice root
- 2g of lightly crushed Poppy seeds
- 1 cup of water

Preparation:
Combine the crushed Poppy seeds with powdered Liquorice, add water, bring to a simmer, and remove from heat. Let it steep for 10 minutes before straining.

Preparation Time: 10 minutes
Dosage: 1 cup, three times a day

Herbal Tea Recipes Whooping Cough

Herbal Remedy for Whooping Cough #1
Ingredients:

- 2 teaspoons chopped Marjoram
- 2 cups boiling water

Preparation Method:
Combine the boiling water with the Marjoram in a container, cover, and allow the mixture to steep for 15 minutes. Strain the tea and allow it to cool to room temperature before drinking.

Preparation time: 15 minutes
Dosage: Drink 1 cup twice daily.

Herbal Remedy for Whooping Cough #2
Ingredients:

- 1-2 teaspoons crushed dried Mullein blossoms
- 1 cup boiling water

Preparation Method:
Add the crushed blossoms to the boiling water, cover, and let the tea steep for 10 minutes. Strain the infusion before drinking.

Preparation time: 10 minutes
Dosage: Drink 1 cup 2-3 times daily.

Herbal Remedy for Whooping Cough #3
Ingredients:

- 2 teaspoons chopped Thyme leaves (tops)
- 1 cup boiling water

Preparation Method:
Steep the chopped Thyme leaves in the boiling water for 10 minutes in a covered container. Strain the tea before consuming.

Preparation time: 10 minutes
Dosage: Drink 1 cup 3-4 times daily.

Recommendation: Thyme tea is also effective for treating spasmodic or dry coughs.

Herbal Remedy for Whooping Cough #4
Ingredients:

- 2/3 teaspoon ground Thyme leaves
- 1/3 teaspoon Sundew whole plant
- 1 cup boiling water

Preparation Method:
Place the herbs in a container, add the boiling water, cover, and steep for 10-15 minutes. Strain the mixture and allow it to cool to room temperature before drinking.

Preparation time: 10-15 minutes
Dosage: Drink 1 cup 2-3 times daily.

Herbal Tea Recipes for Cystitis

Herbal Remedy for Cystitis #1
Ingredients:

- 1-2 teaspoons coarsely powdered Bearberry dried leaves
- 1 cup water

Preparation Method:
Pour the water over the powdered leaves, cover the vessel, and allow it to infuse for 6-12 hours. Avoid heating or boiling the leaves as this can impart bitterness and reduce their effectiveness. Strain the liquid and drink it cold.

Preparation time: 6-12 hours
Dosage: Drink 1 cup twice daily.

Caution: During the course of this treatment, your urine may turn a bright green color. This is harmless. Long-term use is not recommended due to its high tannin content, which may cause constipation or upset stomach.

Herbal Remedy for Cystitis #2
Ingredients:

- 1 teaspoon crushed Birch leaves (fresh or dried)
- 1 cup boiling water

Preparation Method:
Add the Birch leaves to the boiling water, cover, and steep for 5-10 minutes. Strain the infusion and discard the leaves before drinking.

Preparation time: 5-10 minutes
Dosage: Drink 1 cup 3 times daily.

Herbal Remedy for Cystitis #3
Ingredients:

- 1 teaspoon lightly crushed Juniper berries
- 1 cup boiling water

Preparation Method:
Soak the Juniper berries in boiling water for 20 minutes, keeping the container covered. Strain the tea, discard the berries, and drink the infusion morning and evening.

Preparation time: 20 minutes
Dosage: Drink 1 cup twice daily.

Caution: Not recommended for pregnant women or those with kidney inflammation.

Herbal Teas for Diabetes

Herbal Remedy for Diabetes #1
Ingredients:

- 2 tablespoons shredded Babul bark
- 2 cups water

Preparation Method:
Steep the Babul bark in water for 12 hours, keeping the container covered. Strain the tea and drink the liquid.

Preparation time: 12 hours
Dosage: Drink 3-4 tablespoons twice daily.

Herbal Remedy for Diabetes #2
Ingredients:

- 1 teaspoon crushed Jambol seeds
- 1 cup water

Preparation Method:
Soak the Jambol seeds in water for 8 hours, then strain.

Preparation time: 8 hours
Dosage: Drink 1 tablespoon 3 times daily.

Herbal Remedy for Diabetes #3
Ingredients:

- 1 teaspoon crushed Cotton Seed
- 3 cups water

Preparation Method:
Boil the Cotton Seed in a covered container until the water is reduced to 1 cup. Strain the mixture and drink it twice daily.

Preparation time: 30 minutes
Dosage: Drink 1 cup twice daily.

Caution: Not recommended for pregnant women.

Herbal Remedy for Diabetes #4
Ingredients:

- 1-2 teaspoons shredded Dandelion root
- 1 cup water

Preparation Method:
Boil the Dandelion root in water for 2-3 minutes. Remove from heat, cover, and let it steep for 15 minutes. Strain the infusion before drinking.

Preparation time: Boiling time: 2-3 minutes; steeping time: 15 minutes.
Dosage: Drink 1 cup morning and evening for 4-6 weeks.

Herbal Teas for Impotence

Recipe #1

Ingredients:

- 1 teaspoon chopped Coriander leaves
- 1 cup boiling water

Preparation Method:
To prepare the infusion, pour boiling water over the coriander leaves, cover the pan, and let it steep for 15 minutes. Afterward, strain the liquid.

Preparation Time: 15 minutes
Dosage: 2–4 tablespoons per day

Helpful Tip: Coriander leaf extract serves as an aphrodisiac, while the extract from coriander seeds can reduce sexual desire.

Recipe #2

Ingredients:

- 1 tablespoon crushed Marking Nut herb
- ½ cup water

Preparation Method:
Boil the crushed Marking Nut herb in the water until only half of the liquid remains. Strain and discard the herb.

Preparation Time: 3–4 minutes
Dosage: 4 tablespoons per day

Recipe #3

Ingredients:

- Crushed Peepal fruit, root, bark, or tender shoots
- Milk

Preparation Method:
Add the crushed herb to the milk and boil for 10 minutes. Strain the liquid, and sweeten with sugar or honey.

Preparation Time: 10 minutes
Dosage: ¼ cup at bedtime

Herbal Tea Recipes for Indigestion

Herbal Tea Recipes for Indigestion

Recipe #1

Ingredients:

- 1 teaspoon crushed Aniseed seeds
- 1 cup boiling water

Preparation Method:
Pour boiling water over the crushed seeds and let it steep for 3–5 minutes. Strain the tea and drink it cold.

Preparation Time: 3–5 minutes
Dosage: 1–2 cups per day, 1 tablespoon at a time

Recipe #2

Ingredients:

- 1–3 grams Beleric Myrobalan fruit pulp
- 2 cups water

Preparation Method:
Boil the fruit pulp in water for 15 minutes. Strain the extract, discard the fruit, and enjoy your tea.

Preparation Time: 15 minutes
Dosage: 1 cup, twice a day

Recipe #3

Ingredients:

- 3–12 grams powdered Chebulic Myrobalan
- 1 cup water

Preparation Method:
Mix the powdered herb with water. Prepare the tea at room temperature, avoiding any boiling or heating.

Preparation Time: 5 minutes
Dosage: 1 cup, twice a day

Recipe #4

Ingredients:

- 1 teaspoon crushed Cumin seeds

- 2 cups water

Preparation Method:
Add the crushed seeds to water, cover, and boil the mixture for 15 minutes. Strain and drink the tea while it's hot or warm.

Preparation Time: 15 minutes
Dosage: 1–2 cups per day

Recipe #5

Ingredients:

- 30 grams shredded Ginger rhizomes
- 2 cups boiling water

Preparation Method:
Steep the shredded ginger in boiling water for 5–20 minutes in a covered container. Strain and drink the infusion 1–2 times a day.

Preparation Time: 5–20 minutes
Dosage: 1 cup, twice a day

Recipe #6

Ingredients:

- 1 teaspoon crushed Spearmint leaves
- 2 cups water

Preparation Method:
Add the crushed spearmint leaves to water, cover, and bring to a boil. Continue boiling for 15 minutes, then strain and enjoy while the tea is still warm.

Preparation Time: 15 minutes
Dosage: 1 cup, twice a day

Recipe #7

Ingredients:

- 11 grams powdered Cardamom seeds
- 60 grams powdered Coriander seeds
- 3 cups water

Preparation Method:
Combine the cardamom and coriander powders with water. Cover the pan, and simmer until the water reduces by half. Strain and consume the tea.

Preparation Time: 35 minutes
Dosage:
Adults: 3–4 tablespoons, 3 times a day
Children: 3–4 teaspoons, 3 times a day

Herbal Teas for Insomnia

Recipe #1

Ingredients:

- 1–2 teaspoons shredded Valerian root
- 1 cup water

Preparation Method:
Soak the shredded valerian root in water for 8 hours in a covered container. Gently warm the mixture, strain, and drink the filtrate in the evening.

Preparation Time: 8 hours
Dosage: 1 cup in the evening

Caution: This tea is not recommended for pregnant or nursing women.

Recipe #2

Ingredients:

- 1.5 grams Almonds
- 1.5 grams Bitter Bottle Gourd
- 3 grams Poppy seeds
- 1 cup boiling water

Preparation Method:
Crush the almonds, bottle gourd, and poppy seeds into a fine powder. Stir the mixture into the boiling water, then strain. Discard half the liquid and sweeten the remaining half with a bit of sugar. Drink at bedtime.

Preparation Time: 10 minutes
Dosage: ½ cup at bedtime

Recipe #3

Ingredients:

- 1–2 teaspoons crushed California Poppy flower
- 1 cup boiling water

Preparation Method:
Steep the crushed California Poppy flowers in boiling water for 10 minutes. Strain and drink the infusion morning and evening for several weeks.

Preparation Time: 10 minutes
Dosage: 1 cup, twice a day

Recipe #4

Ingredients:

- 1 teaspoon crushed Hops plant
- 1 cup boiling water

Preparation Method:
Soak the hops in boiling water for 15 minutes in a covered pan. Strain and drink in the evening.

Preparation Time: 15 minutes
Dosage: 1 cup in the evening

Recipe #5

Ingredients:

- 1–2 teaspoons crushed Mullein flowers
- 4 cups boiling water

Preparation Method:
Add the mullein flowers to the boiling water, cover, and let the mixture steep for 20 minutes. Strain and enjoy the tea.

Preparation Time: 20 minutes
Dosage: 1 cup, 4 times a day

Herbal Tea Recipes for Jaundice

Recipe #1

Ingredients:

- 1 teaspoon finely chopped Gokulakanta root
- 2 cups water

Preparation Method:
Boil the Gokulakanta root in water for 20–30 minutes in a covered vessel. Strain and consume 2–3 times a day.

Preparation Time: 20–30 minutes
Dosage: 2–4 tablespoons, 2–3 times a day

Recipe #2

Ingredients:

- 1–2 teaspoons granulated Marigold flowers
- 2 cups boiling water

Preparation Method:
Place the marigold flowers in a container, add boiling water, cover, and steep for 15 minutes. Strain and drink once a day.

Preparation Time: 15 minutes
Dosage: 1 cup per day

Recipe #3

Ingredients:

- 35 grams crushed Neem leaves
- ½ cup water
- 12 grams Honey

Preparation Method:
Boil the neem leaves in water until the liquid is reduced by half. Keep the vessel covered while boiling. Strain the concentrate, sweeten with honey, and drink twice a day.

Preparation Time: 3–4 minutes
Dosage: ¼ cup, twice a day

Recipe #4

Ingredients:

- 1–4 grams powdered Peepal bark
- ¼ cup water

Preparation Method:
Combine the powdered peepal bark with water in a pan. Simmer until the liquid is reduced by half, then strain and drink the extract in the morning.

Preparation Time: 2–3 minutes
Dosage: 1 tablespoon per day

Recipe #5

Ingredients:

- 1 teaspoon powdered Picrorhiza seeds
- 1 cup boiling water

Preparation Method:
Mix the powdered seeds with boiling water, cover, and steep for 10–15 minutes. Strain and drink the tea.

Preparation Time: 10–15 minutes
Dosage: ½ cup, twice a day

Recipe #6

Ingredients:

- 1 teaspoon ground Wormwood (fresh or dried)
- 1 cup boiling water

Preparation Method:
Combine the wormwood and boiling water in a covered vessel. Let it stand for 10–15 minutes, then strain and drink after meals.

Preparation Time: 10–15 minutes
Dosage: 1 cup, 3 times a day after meals

Recipe #7

Ingredients:

- 6 grams crushed Fennel seeds
- 6 grams crushed Mint leaves
- 6 grams crushed Rose flowers
- ¾ cup water

Preparation Method:
Boil the fennel, mint, and rose flowers in water. After removing from the heat, cover and allow it to cool to room temperature for 15–20 minutes. Strain the decoction and drink twice a day.

Preparation Time: 15–20 minutes
Dosage: ¾ cup, twice a day

Herbal Teas for Kidney Stones

Herbal Recipe #1 for Kidney Stones
Ingredients:

- 15g Crushed Flax Seeds
- 2 cups Boiling Water

Preparation Method:
Pour the boiling water over the crushed flax seeds. Cover and allow the mixture to steep for 5 minutes for a light tea, or 20 minutes for a stronger brew. Strain the tea before drinking.

Preparation Time: 5-20 minutes.
Dosage: 1-2 cups per day.

Herbal Recipe #2 for Kidney Stones
Ingredients:

- 1-2 teaspoons Fresh, Crushed Juniper Berries
- 1 cup Boiling Water

Preparation Method:
Steep the crushed juniper berries in boiling water for 2 minutes, then strain the mixture.

Preparation Time: 15 minutes.
Dosage: ¼ - 1 oz cup per day.

Herbal Tea Recipe #3 for Kidney Stones
Ingredients:

- ½ - 2 teaspoons Shredded Madder Root
- 1 cup Water

Preparation Method:
Soak the shredded madder root in 1 cup of water for 8 hours in a covered container. Afterward, strain the mixture and discard the root. Drink the remaining liquid twice daily.

Preparation Time: 8 hours.
Dosage: 1 cup, twice a day.
Note: Madder tea may cause urine to turn red, a harmless side effect.

Herbal Recipe #4 for Kidney Stones
Ingredients:

- 1 teaspoon Crushed Parsley Fruit
- 1 ¼ cups Boiling Water

Preparation Method:
Combine the crushed parsley fruit with the boiling water. Cover the mixture and let it steep for 15 minutes before straining.

Preparation Time: 15 minutes.
Dosage: 3 tablespoons per day.
Warning: Pregnant or nursing women should avoid this tea.

Herbal Recipe #5 for Kidney Stones
Ingredients:

- 1 teaspoon Crushed Dried/Fresh Rupturewort
- 1 cup Boiling Water

Preparation Method:
Add the crushed rupturewort to boiling water, cover, and let the mixture steep for 30 minutes. Strain before drinking.

Preparation Time: 30 minutes.
Dosage: 1 cup, three times per day.

Herbal Tea Recipe #6 for Kidney Stones
Ingredients:

- 2 teaspoons Crushed Violet Leaves
- 1 cup Water

Preparation Method:
Pour boiling water over the crushed violet leaves. Cover and allow the mixture to steep for 24 hours. Strain and discard the leaves.

Preparation Time: 24 hours.
Dosage: 1 cup, twice a day.

Herbal Recipe #7 for Kidney Stones
Ingredients:

- 6g Horsegram
- 1½ tablespoons Grated Radish
- ½ cup Water

Preparation Method:
Boil the horsegram in ½ cup of water for 2-3 minutes. Remove from heat, strain the tea, and add the squeezed extract from the grated radish.

Preparation Time: 15 minutes.
Dosage: ½ cup in the morning.

Herbal Recipes for Lactation Disorders

Herbal Recipe #1 for Lactation Disorders
Ingredients:

- 1 teaspoon Crushed Aniseed
- 1 cup Boiling Water

Preparation Method:
Soak the crushed aniseed in boiling water for 3-5 minutes. Strain the tea and allow it to cool completely before drinking.

Preparation Time: 3-5 minutes.
Dosage: 1 cup, twice a day, 1 teaspoon at a time.

Herbal Recipe #2 for Lactation Disorders
Ingredients:

- 1.5-3g Crushed Black Cumin Seeds
- ¼ cup Water

Preparation Method:
Grind the black cumin seeds in ¼ cup of water using a mortar and pestle. Strain the mixture and sweeten the liquid extract with honey to taste.

Preparation Time: 5 minutes.
Dosage: ¼ cup per day.

Herbal Recipe #3 for Lactation Disorders
Ingredients:

- 6g Crushed Nut Grass Tubers
- 4 cups Water

Preparation Method:
Cook the crushed nut grass tubers in 4 cups of water for 15 minutes in a covered container. Strain the decoction and drink the liquid.

Preparation Time: 15 minutes.
Dosage: 1 cup, four times a day.

Herbal Tea Recipe #4 for Lactation Disorders
Ingredients:

- ¼ - ½ teaspoon Aniseed
- ½ - 1 teaspoon Caraway Seeds
- ¼ - ½ teaspoon Fennel Seeds
- 1 cup Water

Preparation Method:
Combine the aniseed, caraway, and fennel seeds to make a 1-2 teaspoon herbal mixture. Lightly crush the mixture in a mortar. Add 1 cup of water and heat until the water begins to simmer. Remove from heat and cover the tea to steep for an additional 10 minutes. Strain before drinking.

Preparation Time: 10 minutes.
Dosage: 1 cup per day.

Herbal Tea Recipe #5 for Lactation Disorders
Ingredients:

- ¾ teaspoon Lightly Crushed Aniseed
- 1¼ teaspoons Lightly Crushed Fenugreek Seeds
- 1 cup Water

Preparation Method:
Simmer the aniseed and fenugreek seeds in water, then remove from heat. Cover the tea and let it steep for 10 minutes. Strain and serve.

Preparation Time: 10 minutes.
Dosage: 1 cup, three times a day.

Herbal Teas for Laryngitis

Herbal Tea #1 for Laryngitis
Ingredients:

- 1-2 teaspoons Shredded Caraway Root
- 1 cup Water

Preparation Method:
Simmer the shredded caraway root and water in a covered container. Once the mixture reaches a simmer, remove it from the heat and let it steep for 15-20 minutes. Strain and your tea is ready to drink.

Preparation Time: 15-20 minutes.
Dosage: 1 cup, twice a day.

Herbal Tea Recipe #2 for Laryngitis
Ingredients:

- 2 teaspoons Chopped Whole Hedge Mustard Plant
- ½ cup Boiling Water

Preparation Method:
Combine the chopped hedge mustard and boiling water in a covered container. Let the mixture steep for 20 minutes before straining.

Preparation Time: 20 minutes.
Dosage: ½ cup, twice a day.

Herbal Recipe #3 for Laryngitis
Ingredients:

- 12g Crushed Linseed
- 1 cup Water

Preparation Method:
Combine the crushed linseed and water, then bring the mixture to a boil. Reduce the liquid by half through simmering. Strain the tea and add a touch of honey to taste.

Preparation Time: 7-8 minutes.
Dosage: 1 cup, twice a day.

Homemade Herbal Tea Recipe #4 for Laryngitis
Ingredients:

- 1 teaspoon Shredded Wild Ginger Root
- 1 cup Water

Preparation Method:
Combine the shredded wild ginger root and water in a covered container. Gently bring the mixture to a simmer, then remove from the heat and let it steep for 15 minutes. Strain and allow the tea to cool to room temperature before drinking.

Preparation Time: 15 minutes.
Dosage: 1 cup, twice a day.

Herbal Teas for Leucorrhoea

Homemade Herbal Recipe for Leucorrhoea #1
Ingredients:

- 2 teaspoons Crushed Fenugreek Seeds
- 4 cups Water

Preparation Method:
Combine the fenugreek seeds with the water and heat the mixture over a low flame until it reaches a simmer. Let the tea simmer for 30 minutes. Once cooled to room temperature, strain the tea.

Preparation Time: 30 minutes.
Dosage: 1 cup, four times a day.

Herbal Tea for Leucorrhoea #2
Ingredients:

- 1 teaspoon Powdered Hazardana Herb
- 1 cup Water

Preparation Method:
Stir the powdered herb into 1 cup of water. Cover and let the mixture sit overnight. Strain the tea the following morning.

Preparation Time: 8-10 hours.
Dosage: 1 cup per day.

Herbal Tea Recipes for Menstrual Disorders

Herbal Tea Recipe for Menstrual Disorders #1
Ingredients:

- 15g Crushed Dried Asoka Bark
- 1 cup Water

Preparation Method:
Add the water to the crushed asoka bark and bring the mixture to a boil. Continue boiling until the liquid is reduced to ¼ cup. Remove from heat and allow to cool. Strain and sweeten with sugar or honey.

Preparation Time: 10 minutes.
Dosage: 1-4 tablespoons per day.

Recommendation: For fresh bark, use only ½ cup water and reduce it by boiling to 2 tablespoons. This tea helps alleviate excessive menstruation.

Herbal Tea for Menstrual Disorders #2
Ingredients:

- 1 teaspoon Powdered Black Cumin Seeds
- 1 cup Boiling Water

Preparation Method:
Add the powdered black cumin to 1 cup of boiling water. Cover and let the tea steep for 15 minutes. Strain and serve.

Preparation Time: 15 minutes.
Dosage: ¼ cup, twice a day.

Recommendation: This tea supports menstrual flow.

Herbal Recipe for Menstrual Disorders #3
Ingredients:

- 1-2 teaspoons Granulated Marigold Flowers
- 1 cup Boiling Water

Preparation Method:
Steep the granulated marigold flowers in boiling water in a covered container for 15 minutes. Strain the liquid and discard the flowers.

Preparation Time: 15 minutes.
Dosage: 1 cup per day.

Herbal Tea Recipe for Menstrual Disorders #4
Ingredients:

- 12g Crushed Pomegranate Bark
- 1 cup Water

Preparation Method:
Simmer the crushed pomegranate bark in 1 cup of water until only half the water remains. Strain the decoction and drink in the morning.

Preparation Time: 7-8 minutes.
Dosage: ½ cup in the morning.

Recommendation: This tea helps control excessive bleeding during menstruation.

Herbal Teas for Menstrual Disorders #5
Ingredients:

- 6g Powdered Embelia Plant
- 6g Powdered Dried Ginger
- 1 ¾ cups Water
- 6g Sugar

Preparation Method:
Combine the powdered embelia and ginger in the water. Boil for 15 minutes, then remove from heat. Strain the tea and sweeten with sugar.

Preparation Time: 15 minutes.
Dosage: ¾ cup per day.

Recommendation: This tea relieves painful menstruation.

Herbal Tea Recipes for Menstrual Disorders #6
Ingredients:

- 6g Crushed Juniper Berries
- 6g Crushed Myrrh
- 1 ½ cups Water

Preparation Method:
Boil the juniper berries and myrrh in water for 15 minutes in a covered container. Strain and drink in the morning.

Preparation Time: 15 minutes.
Dosage: ½ cup in the morning for 10 days.

Recommendation: This tea is ideal for women experiencing painful menstruation.

Herbal Tea Recipes for Nausea

Homemade Herbal Recipe for Nausea #1
Ingredients:

- Crushed Black Pepper Seeds

Preparation Method:
Combine the crushed black pepper seeds with water and bring to a simmer. Remove from heat, cover, and let it stand for 10 minutes before straining the decoction.

Preparation Time: 10 minutes
Dosage: 10-30 drops per day
Note: Adjust the dosage for children according to their age.

Herbal Recipe for Nausea #2
Ingredients:

- 1-2 teaspoons Crushed Peppermint Leaves
- 1 cup Boiling Water

Preparation Method:
Place the crushed peppermint leaves in a covered vessel and pour the boiling water over them. Let the tea steep for 10 minutes, then strain and drink while hot.

Preparation Time: 10 minutes
Dosage: 1-2 cups per day

Herbal Tea for Nausea #3
Ingredients:

- 1 teaspoon Crushed Spearmint Leaves
- 2 cups Water

Preparation Method:
Bring the water and crushed spearmint leaves to a boil, then remove from heat and let it steep, covered, for 10-15 minutes. Strain the tea, discarding the leaves.

Preparation Time: 10-15 minutes
Dosage: 1 cup, three times a day

Herbal Tea Recipe for Nausea #4
Ingredients:

- 2/3 teaspoon Ground Balm Leaves
- 2/3 teaspoon Ground Chamomile Blossoms
- 2/3 teaspoon Ground Peppermint Leaves
- 1 cup Boiling Water

Preparation Method:
Mix the three ground herbs in a container, pour boiling water over the mixture, cover, and let it brew for 10 minutes. Strain and sip the tea while it's still hot.

Preparation Time: 10 minutes
Dosage: 1-2 cups per day

Herbal Recipe for Nausea #5
Ingredients:

- 1/3 teaspoon Ground Black Horehound Plant
- 1/3 teaspoon Ground Java Galangal Plant
- 1/3 teaspoon Ground Marshmallow Plant
- 1 cup Boiling Water

Preparation Method:
Add the ground herbs to boiling water, cover, and let it stand for 15 minutes. Strain and drink.

Preparation Time: 15 minutes
Dosage: 1 cup, three times a day

Herbal Teas for Nervous Exhaustion

Homemade Herbal Tea Recipe for Nervous Exhaustion #1
Ingredients:

- ½ teaspoon Shredded American Ginseng Root
- 1 cup Water

Preparation Method:
Boil the shredded ginseng root in water for 1 minute, then cover and let it steep for 15 minutes. Strain and drink.

Preparation Time: 1 minute boiling, 15 minutes steeping
Dosage: 1-2 cups per day

Herbal Recipe for Nervous Exhaustion #2
Ingredients:

- 1 teaspoon Crushed Rosemary Leaves

- 1 cup Boiling Water

Preparation Method:
Immerse the crushed rosemary leaves in the boiling water. Cover and steep for 15 minutes, then strain the tea and drink.

Preparation Time: 15 minutes
Dosage: 1 cup, twice a day

Herbal Tea for Nervous Exhaustion #3
Ingredients:

- ½ teaspoon Crushed Lavender Blossoms
- ½ teaspoon Crushed Rosemary Leaves
- 1 cup Boiling Water

Preparation Method:
Place the herbs in a pan, pour boiling water over them, and cover. Let it brew for 10 minutes, then strain and discard the herbs.

Preparation Time: 15 minutes
Dosage: 1 cup per day

Herbal Tea Recipes for Neuralgia

Herbal Recipe for Neuralgia #1
Ingredients:

- 10g Hops Herb
- 2 cups Boiling Water

Preparation Method:
Steep the hops in the boiling water for 15 minutes in a covered container. Strain and drink.

Preparation Time: 15 minutes
Dosage: 1 cup, twice a day

Homemade Herbal Recipe for Neuralgia #2
Ingredients:

- 1 teaspoon Powdered Valerian Rhizomes/Root
- 1 cup Boiling Water

Preparation Method:
Steep the powdered valerian in boiling water for 10 minutes, keeping the pan covered. Strain and discard the herb.

Preparation Time: 10 minutes
Dosage: ¼ cup, four times a day
Note: Not recommended for pregnant or nursing women.

Herbal Tea for Neuralgia #3
Ingredients:

- 1 teaspoon Shredded Willow Bark
- 2 cups Water

Preparation Method:
Boil the shredded willow bark in 2 cups of water for 15 minutes in a covered vessel. Remove from heat and strain the decoction.

Preparation Time: 15 minutes
Dosage: 1 cup, twice a day

Herbal Tea Recipes for Dropsy

Herbal Recipe for Dropsy #1
Ingredients:

- 1-2 teaspoons Finely Chopped Elecampane Root
- 2 cups Water

Preparation Method:
Boil the chopped elecampane root for 2-3 minutes, then remove from heat and let it steep for 15 minutes. Strain and drink.

Preparation Time: 2-3 minutes boiling, 15 minutes steeping
Dosage: 1 cup, twice a day

Homemade Herbal Tea Recipe for Dropsy #2
Ingredients:

- 2 teaspoons Chopped Germander Flowering Plant
- 2 cups Boiling Water

Preparation Method:
Combine the germander and boiling water in a covered container. Let it steep for 15 minutes, then strain and drink.

Preparation Time: 15 minutes
Dosage: 1 cup, twice a day

Herbal Recipe for Dropsy #3
Ingredients:

- 30g Lightly Pounded Gokulakanta Root
- 2 ½ cups Water

Preparation Method:
Boil the gokulakanta root in 2 ½ cups water until the volume is reduced to 1 ½ cups (about 15-20 minutes). Keep the vessel covered throughout. After cooking, cool, strain, and drink.

Preparation Time: 15-20 minutes
Dosage: 2-4 tablespoons every 2 hours

Herbal Tea for Dropsy #4
Ingredients:

- 1 teaspoon Chopped Dried Bean Pods (without seeds)
- 1 cup Water

Preparation Method:
Boil the chopped bean pods in water for 2-3 minutes, then remove from heat, cover, and let it stand for 15 minutes. Strain and drink.

Preparation Time: 2-3 minutes boiling, 15 minutes steeping
Dosage: 1 cup, twice a day

Herbal Recipe for Dropsy #5
Ingredients:

- 1 teaspoon Ground Parsley Plant (including seeds and root)
- 1 cup Water

Preparation Method:
Simmer the parsley in water for 2-3 minutes, then remove from heat and cover for 15 minutes to steep. Strain and drink.

Preparation Time: 2-3 minutes boiling, 15 minutes steeping
Dosage: 1 cup, twice a day
Note: Not recommended for pregnant or nursing women.

Herbal Tea Recipes for Phlebitis & Varicose Veins

Recipe #1: Rue Herb Tea
Ingredients:

- 2 teaspoons Rue herb, chopped
- 1 cup boiling water

Preparation Method:
Place the chopped Rue herb into the boiling water and cover the vessel. Let it steep for 15 minutes. Strain and drink the tea as recommended.
Preparation Time: 15 minutes
Dosage: 1 cup, 3 times a day

Recipe #2: Yellow Sweet Clover Tea
Ingredients:

- 2 teaspoons Yellow Sweet Clover herb, chopped
- 1 cup boiling water

Preparation Method:
Place the chopped Yellow Sweet Clover into a covered container. Pour the boiling water over it, close the lid, and allow the tea to brew for 10 minutes. Strain and enjoy.
Preparation Time: 10 minutes
Dosage: 1 cup, 3-4 times a day

Herbal Tea Recipes for Piles

Recipe #1: Mullein Leaf Tea
Ingredients:

- 1 teaspoon Mullein leaves, crushed
- 1 cup boiling water

Preparation Method:
Add the crushed Mullein leaves to the boiling water and cover the vessel. Let it steep for 20 minutes, then strain and drink the tea.
Preparation Time: 20 minutes
Dosage: 1-2 cups a day, 1 tablespoon at a time

Recipe #2: Smartweed Tea
Ingredients:

- 2-3 teaspoons Smartweed herb (dried or fresh), crushed
- 1 cup water

Preparation Method:
Combine the Smartweed with the water and heat until it reaches a simmer. Remove from heat, cover, and let it sit for 15 minutes. Strain and drink.
Preparation Time: 15 minutes
Dosage: 1 cup, twice a day (morning and evening)

Recipe #3: Witch Hazel Tea
Ingredients:

- 1 teaspoon Witch Hazel leaves/bark, crushed
- 1 cup boiling water

Preparation Method:
Boil the Witch Hazel in water for 2-3 minutes. Remove from heat, cover, and let the mixture sit for 10 minutes. Strain and drink.

Preparation Time: 2-3 minutes boiling, 10 minutes standing
Dosage: 1 cup, twice a day (morning and evening)

Recipe #4: Yarrow Herb Tea
Ingredients:

- 1-2 teaspoons Yarrow herb or blossoms, crushed
- 1 cup water

Preparation Method:
Place the Yarrow in a covered container, pour water over it, and let it steep for 5-6 hours. Strain and drink.
Preparation Time: 5-6 hours
Dosage: 1 cup, twice a day

Recipe #5: Hops & Valerian Root Tea
Ingredients:

- ½ teaspoon Hops, crushed
- ½ teaspoon Valerian root, crushed
- 1 cup water

Preparation Method:
Add the crushed herbs to the water and cover the vessel. Let the mixture sit for 8 hours, shaking the container occasionally. Strain and serve.
Preparation Time: 8 hours
Dosage: 1 cup, twice a day

Note: Not recommended for pregnant or nursing women.

Herbal Tea Recipes for Enlarged Prostate Gland

Recipe: Stinging Nettle Root Tea
Ingredients:

- 1 teaspoon Stinging Nettle root, powdered
- 1 ¼ cups water

Preparation Method:
Boil the powdered Stinging Nettle root in water for 15 minutes. Remove from heat and let it sit for another 15 minutes.
Preparation Time: 15 minutes boiling, 15 minutes standing
Dosage: 2-3 teaspoons a day

Herbal Tea Recipes for Rheumatism

Recipe #1: Ash Leaves Tea
Ingredients:

- 2-3 teaspoons Ash leaves, chopped
- 2 cups water

Preparation Method:
Boil the Ash leaves and water for 10 minutes. Remove from heat, cover, and let the mixture stand for another 10 minutes. Strain and drink.
Preparation Time: 10 minutes boiling, 10 minutes standing
Dosage: 1 cup, twice a day

Recipe #2: Bittersweet Twigs Tea
Ingredients:

- 30g Bittersweet twigs, chopped
- 3 cups water

Preparation Method:
Cook the twigs in water until the liquid reduces to 1 ½ cups. Strain and drink.
Preparation Time: 20 minutes
Dosage: 1 ½ cups, 3 times a day

Recipe #3: Couch Grass Rhizomes Tea
Ingredients:

- 1-2 teaspoons Couch Grass rhizomes, chopped
- 4 cups water

Preparation Method:
Combine the Couch Grass rhizomes and water. Bring to a boil, then cover and simmer for 10 minutes. Let the mixture stand for 30 minutes. Strain and drink.
Preparation Time: 10 minutes boiling, 30 minutes standing
Dosage: 1 cup, 4 times a day

Recipe #4: Dandelion Leaves Tea
Ingredients:

- 1-2 teaspoons Dandelion leaves, shredded
- 1 cup water

Preparation Method:
Boil the Dandelion leaves in water for 1 minute. Remove from heat, cover, and let it sit for 15 minutes. Strain and drink.
Preparation Time: 1 minute boiling, 15 minutes standing
Dosage: 1 cup, morning and evening for 4-8 weeks, especially during the spring and winter months

---

Recipe #5: Parsley Tea
Ingredients:

- 1 handful Parsley plant with stem, chopped
- 3 cups water

Preparation Method:
Add the Parsley to the water and bring to a boil. Reduce the heat, cover, and simmer for 30 minutes. Strain and drink.
Preparation Time: 30 minutes
Dosage: 1 cup, twice a day

Caution: Not recommended for pregnant or nursing women.

Recipe #6: Stinging Nettle Tea
Ingredients:

- 1-2 teaspoons Stinging Nettle leaves, dried and crushed
- 1 cup water

Preparation Method:
Place the Stinging Nettle leaves in the water and bring to a boil. Boil for 2 minutes, then cover and let it cool for 15 minutes. Strain and drink.
Preparation Time: 2 minutes boiling, 15 minutes standing
Dosage: 1 cup, twice a day for 4-6 weeks, 2-3 times a year

Recipe #7: Willow Bark Tea
Ingredients:

- 2-3 teaspoons Willow bark, crushed
- 4 cups water

Preparation Method:
Boil the Willow bark for 5 minutes. Cover, remove from heat, and let it sit for 15 minutes. Once it has cooled, strain and drink.
Preparation Time: 5 minutes boiling, 15 minutes standing
Dosage: 1 cup, twice a day

Herbal Teas for Skin Disorders

Recipe #1: English Walnut Tea
Ingredients:

- 2 teaspoons English Walnut meat and dried leaves, crushed
- 1 cup water

Preparation Method:
Soak the crushed walnut meat and leaves in water for 5-10 minutes. Strain and drink.
Preparation Time: 5-10 minutes
Dosage: 1 cup, twice a day for several weeks

Note: Effective for eczema or dermatitis.

Recipe #2: Neem Leaf Tea
Ingredients:

- 2 tablespoons Neem leaves, crushed
- 2 cups water

Preparation Method:
Add the crushed Neem leaves to water and bring to a boil in a covered container. Boil for 15 minutes, then strain. You may add sugar or honey if desired.
Preparation Time: 15 minutes
Dosage: ¼ - ½ cup, 4 times a day

Note: Excellent for skin diseases, including boils.

Herbal Tea Recipes for Blood in the Urine

Recipe #1: Barley Seed Tea
Ingredients:

- 25g Barley seeds, crushed
- 4 cups water

Preparation Method:
Combine the crushed barley seeds with the water in a pan, cover, and bring to a boil. Allow it to simmer for 20 minutes. Strain and enjoy as directed.
Preparation Time: 20 minutes
Dosage: 1 cup, 3 times a day

Recipe #2: Vasaka Leaf Tea
Ingredients:

- 12g Vasaka leaves
- 1 cup water

Preparation Method:
Grind the Vasaka leaves in the water, then strain the liquid. Drink the strained infusion.
Preparation Time: 5 minutes
Dosage: 1 cup, twice a day

Herbal Tea Recipes for Painful Urination (Dysuria)

Recipe #1: Flax Seed Tea
Ingredients:

- 15g Flax seeds, crushed
- 2 cups water

Preparation Method:
Soak the crushed flax seeds in water for 5-20 minutes in a covered pan. Strain and drink the tea, either hot or warm.
Preparation Time: 5 minutes for light tea, 20 minutes for stronger tea
Dosage: 1-2 cups a day

Recipe #2: Goldenrod Tea
Ingredients:

- 1-2 teaspoons Goldenrod (whole plant), ground
- 4 cups water

Preparation Method:
Bring the Goldenrod and water to a boil in a covered pan for 2 minutes. Remove from heat and let it cool for 10-15 minutes. Strain and drink.
Preparation Time: 2 minutes boiling, 10-15 minutes standing
Dosage: 1 cup, 2-4 times a day

Recipe #3: Onion Bulb Tea
Ingredients:

- 6g Onion bulbs, crushed
- 2 cups water

Preparation Method:
Combine the crushed onion bulbs with water and bring to a boil. Continue boiling until the water is reduced to 1 cup. Allow the decoction to cool, then strain and drink.
Preparation Time: 15 minutes
Dosage: 1 cup, twice a day

Recipe #4: Purslane Leaf Tea
Ingredients:

- 1 teaspoon Purslane leaves, crushed
- ½ cup boiling water

Preparation Method:
Steep the crushed Purslane leaves in boiling water in a covered pan for 12 hours. Strain the infusion, discard the leaves, and drink 1 ½ teaspoons of the remaining extract twice a day.
Preparation Time: 12 hours
Dosage: 1 ½ teaspoons, twice a day

Recipe #5: Senna Leaf Tea
Ingredients:

- 10-30g Senna leaves, finely chopped or powdered
- 4 cups water

Preparation Method:
Pour the water over the Senna leaves and let the mixture stand for 5-6 hours. Strain and drink.
Preparation Time: 5-6 hours
Dosage: 1 cup, 4 times a day

Herbal Tea Recipes for Vomiting

Recipe #1: Chamomile & Herb Tea
Ingredients:

- ½ teaspoon Chamomile flowers, ground
- ½ teaspoon European Centaury, ground
- ½ teaspoon Fennel seeds, crushed
- ½ teaspoon Lemon balm, ground
- ½ teaspoon Peppermint, ground
- 1 cup hot water

Preparation Method:
Combine all the herbs and pour hot water over them. Cover the pan and let it steep for 15 minutes. Strain and drink the tea.
Preparation Time: 15 minutes
Dosage: 1 cup, twice a day

Caution: Not recommended for children under two years of age.

Recipe #2: Chamomile & Mint Tea
Ingredients:

- ½ teaspoon Chamomile flowers, ground
- ½ teaspoon European Centaury, ground
- ½ teaspoon Peppermint, ground
- ½ teaspoon Spearmint, ground
- 1 teaspoon Wormwood, ground
- 1 cup boiling water

Preparation Method:
Combine all the herbs and pour boiling water over them. Cover the pan and let it steep for 15 minutes. Strain the infusion and discard the herbs.
Preparation Time: 15 minutes
Dosage: 1 cup, 3 times a day

Recipe #3: Black Horehound & Chamomile Tea
Ingredients:

- 1/3 teaspoon Black horehound, ground
- 1/3 teaspoon Chamomile flowers, ground
- 1/3 teaspoon Meadowsweet, ground
- 1 cup boiling water

Preparation Method:
Combine the herbs in boiling water and let them steep for 15 minutes. Strain and drink.

Preparation Time: 15 minutes
Dosage: 1 cup, twice a day

Recommendation: This tea is effective for controlling vomiting during pregnancy.

Herbal Tea Recipes for Wounds

Recipe #1: Lemon Fruit Tea
Ingredients:

- 1 lemon, halved
- 2 cups water

Preparation Method:
Cover the halved lemon with water in a pan and bring it to a boil. Let it boil for 15 minutes, then remove from heat. Allow it to sit for an additional 10 minutes. Strain and drink.
Preparation Time: 15 minutes boiling, 10 minutes standing
Dosage: 1 cup a day

Recipe #2: Turmeric & Alum Milk Tea
Ingredients:

- 3g Turmeric powder
- ½g Alum powder
- ½ cup cow's milk

Preparation Method:
Mix the turmeric and alum with milk, then heat the mixture to about 70°C. Drink as recommended.
Preparation Time: 5 minutes
Dosage: ½ cup a day for several days

Recipe #3: Stinging Nettle Tea for Wounds
Ingredients:

- 2 teaspoons Stinging Nettle leaves, dried and crushed
- 1 cup water

Preparation Method:
Boil the Stinging Nettle leaves in water for 5 minutes. Remove from heat, cover the pan, and let it stand for 1 hour. Strain and drink.
Preparation Time: 5 minutes boiling, 1 hour standing
Dosage: 1/3 cup, 3 times a day